H

RAISE YOUR TODDLER

Learn how to improve your toddler's behavior during his growth processes positively.

MARLA CALLORY

within this document, including, but not limited to, — errors, omissions, or inaccuracies.

Table of Contents

INTRODUCTION 8

CHAPTER 1: THE MONTESSORI METHOD 12

WHAT IS THE MONTESSORI METHOD? 12
A SHORT HISTORY OF THE MONTESSORI METHOD 13
PRINCIPLES OF MONTESSORI PHILOSOPHY 14
Self-Actualization through Montessori Method 14
The display of mutual work and integrity 15
Holistic Development of Students 16
The thriving layers of Positivity through Montessori method 17
Individualism in a child 18
Creation of well-structured routines 18
HOW LIBERTY IS ACCESSED IN THE CHILD'S MIND THROUGH THE MONTESSORI METHODS .. 20

CHAPTER 2: TODDLER MENTAL DEVELOPMENT 23

STAGES OF MENTAL DEVELOPMENT: 24
From Birth to Three Years: 24
From Three to Six Years: 24
Later Childhood: 24
THE VARIOUS ASPECTS OF MENTAL DEVELOPMENT: 25
Sensation and Perception: 25
Concept Formation: 26
HOW TO IMPROVE CHILDREN'S MENTAL HEALTH? 30
Pay Attention to Your Psychological Health 30
Build Trust 31
Foster Healthy Relationships with Others 31
Be Reliable 32
Teach Your Child Healthy Ways to Manage Stress 32
Establish Healthy Habits 33
Develop Self-Esteem 33
Provide Possibilities for Independence. 33
Help Your Baby Develop Wholesome Self-Speak. 34
Encourage Your Infant to Expand New Abilities 34
Be the Perfect Model. 34
Play Together 34
GROWTH IN THINKING AND PROBLEM SOLVING: 35

THE GROWTH OF INTELLIGENCE OR INTELLECTUAL DEVELOPMENT: 36

CHAPTER 3: PHYSICAL DEVELOPMENTS OF A TODDLER 41

TODDLER DEVELOPMENTAL MILESTONES 41

12 Months 41

15 Months 42

18 Months 42

2 Years 43

2 ½ Years 44

3 Years 45

GROSS MOTOR DEVELOPMENT 47

FINE MOTOR DEVELOPMENT 47

SIGNS OF DEVELOPMENTAL ISSUES 47

Ages 1–2 Years 48

Ages 2–3 Years 48

PHYSICAL APPEARANCES OF A TODDLER 48

CHAPTER 4: APPLYING THE MONTESSORI METHOD AT HOME 53

PREPARE THE ENVIRONMENT 54

Plan all the materials and activities to include in your child's environment 54

Focus on life skills 55

Help your child learn concentration and inner motivation 56

Take on the role of a Montessori teacher 56

CHAPTER 5: TEACH COOPERATION 59

WAYS TO BE COOPERATIVE WITH THE KIDS 59

Taking turns 59

Explain your reasons for limits and reasons 60

Take time to problem solve 60

Do chores together start at an early age! 61

Giving more praise for cooperative efforts 61

Always be suggestive 62

Give your child choices while maintaining the rules 62

Talk your child about their feelings and let them know yours 63

Explain them the situations in a calm manner 63

Play games with them 63

Always ask permissions before joining 64

Sharing is caring 64

CHAPTER 6: KIND-MINDED PARENTING........ 67

MONTESSORI AT HOME AND MONTESSORI PARENTING........ 68

TODDLERS COMMUNICATION........ 68

What You Can Do........ *69*

Speak Positively, But Praise the Effort More Than the Child........ *72*

CHAPTER 7: ART AND CRAFT ACTIVITIES........ 75

DRAWING........ 76

WATERCOLOR PAINTING........ 77

CUTTING........ 77

SEWING........ 78

PRICK WORK........ 79

PUNCHES........ 79

GLUING........ 80

MODELING CLAY........ 80

COLOR COLLAGE........ 81

MAKING A COLOR BOOKLET........ 82

HANDPRINT FALL TREE CRAFT........ 82

PAPER SHAPE COLLAGE........ 83

CREATING PAPER PLATE ANIMALS........ 83

STICKER WORD ACTIVITY........ 83

COLORED STRAW NECKLACE........ 83

SQUIRT GUN PAINTING........ 84

PALM PAINTING........ 84

MAKING PAPER RAINBOW........ 84

SPRAY PAINT CRAFT........ 85

CHAPTER 8: MOVEMENT THE MONTESSORI WAY........ 87

FREE MOVEMENT AND SENSORY EXPLORATION........ 87

The environment is suitable for the child's height and size......... *88*

Purposeful "Movement" Work........ *88*

Integration of Montessori Materials........ *88*

BENEFITS OF FINE AND GROSS MOTOR SKILLS........ 89

Benefits of fine motor skills........ *89*

Benefits of gross motor skills........ *90*

LEARNING THROUGH PLAY........ 90

HERE ARE SOME WAYS YOUR CHILD CAN DEVELOP MOTOR SKILLS THROUGH PLAYING:........ 93

For the Newborn........ *93*

For the Toddler *95*

CHAPTER 9: HOW TO CREATE A MONTESSORI ENVIRONMENT AT HOME **97**

SIMPLIFY THE ENVIRONMENT 97
EVERYTHING HAS ITS OWN PLACE 98
OPEN SPACES 98
ACCESSIBLE 99
INCORPORATE NATURE 99
CAREFULLY CHOOSE THE TOYS 99
COZY 100

CHAPTER 10: TODDLING **102**

THE BRAIN DEVELOPMENT OF A TODDLER 103
THINGS THAT WILL SCREW UP A TODDLER 104
THE MINI-ADULT THINKING 104
OVERSTIMULATION 105
THINGS THAT WON'T SCREW UP A TODDLER 106
Saying No *107*
Discipline *108*
Not giving a constant barrage of choices *109*
Delayed Gratification *110*

CHAPTER 11: COMMON PARENTING MISTAKES WHEN TRAINING TODDLERS **112**

DISTORTING THE ROUTINE 112
USING A METHOD OF COERCION 112
Modest Method of Coercion *113*
RIGIDLY REBUKING YOUR TODDLER'S MISTAKES 115

CONCLUSION **117**

INTRODUCTION

Every parent wants the best for their children. Children are the apples of their parent's eyes, and parents can't seem to get enough of their cuteness. The way they walk, make up their vocabulary and do things win their hearts and leave them feeling proud of having created something so beautiful. Yes, parents, we are talking to you!

Subjects in the Montessori system and Montessori-specific lessons and exercises are mentioned in detail to help provide a distinctive guideline to the parents and teachers alike to raise their toddlers at home, the Montessori way. The role of the parent and the importance of educating the toddlers as preparation for life are essential ingredients to ensure their proper development and enhancement as makers of men.

This is where a child's development milestones come into play. Child development milestones aim to make parenting for expecting and new parents slightly easier as they set certain parameters of how much a child should develop in a certain timeframe. Think of it as a professional coach's way of timing their best athlete's running performance. They have to hit a few milestones to ensure a solid win. The same is the case with child developmental milestones.

Growth and development don't just entail visible changes in their appearance, weight, or height; it also includes milestones like emotional and social regulation, personality formation, communicating and speaking abilities, and sensory awareness.

Since every child is unique, one mustn't rely too much on these developmental milestones. Instead, look at them as a helpful reminder of what is considered appropriate for what age range. This is essential as many new moms get stressed when they notice that another child the same age is more active than theirs or that their child lacks the cognitive ability to make sense of things around them. Understanding milestones can go a long way in relieving anxiety.

Are you ready to scale up your parenting skills? Read on!

Chapter 1: The Montessori Method

What is the Montessori method?

This is an alternative approach to child education. It was developed using careful, scientific observations of children and their learning needs. These observations were scientifically evaluated and integrated into what is known today as the Montessori method.

Dr. Montessori observed that standard teaching methods fought the very nature of children instead of working with it the response was developing a method that designed an environment of based on children's natural state.

This method is meant to educate children with a more personally adaptive approach. It aims to recognize the child's nature and use that as basis for designing the most suitable learning approach.

For example, it is part of a child's nature to move a lot. Motion creates greater sensory stimulation that lets the child learn more and participate more actively in the learning process. The Montessori method allows children to utilize this nature and that helps them learn more -- by letting them work on the floor with a comfortable mat. That's an entirely different approach than standard education in which educators spend considerable effort and time in keeping children in their seats and force them to do nothing but listen.

A Short History of the Montessori Method

The fact that there are entire schools devoted to Montessori instruction does not mean that Montessori techniques can only be practiced in an institution. In fact, Montessori philosophies are among some of the easiest to implement in your home based on how natural they are to your child. All that you really need to begin your Montessori home school is an understanding of the basic Montessori principles. At the most basic level, Dr. Maria Montessori recognized the following principles as being essential to the development of the young child:

Movement and use of the senses are closely related to cognition and understanding.

Even the youngest of children thrive when they are allowed to maintain some control over their own lives. A child that is given some choice in their education is more likely to comprehend and retain the information learned.

Young children, as well as adults, learn better when they are engaged in an activity that they enjoy. By providing children with activities that they find stimulating, a love of learning is fostered.

External rewards such as certificates and trophies do not supply the same amount of satisfaction as self-respect and a sense of pride. For these reasons, awards for behavior and accomplishments should be reduced.

Learning is best done when the environment suits what is being learned. This point alone makes Montessori perfect for the home environment.

We learn from each other.

How the educator interacts with the child influences the outcome. The educator, or parent in this case, is more of a guide or director rather than an authoritative figure.

Everything has a place. That includes physical objects as well as our thoughts. When a child works in a clean, clear environment that makes sense to their activity, they are better able to retain the knowledge gained.

Principles of Montessori Philosophy

Following are the principles of Montessori Philosophy, which need to be applied in all possible ways.

Self-Actualization through Montessori Method

Let us define the principle of self-actualization first. This is the ability of the child to actualize all their potential their-self or with the help of a parent. The parent must be potent and caring enough that he regularly boosts the child to be patient and learn more. This can be demonstrated through a Montessori principle that the child is given a playground. The father observes more of the child's work and when he sees them getting down, then the father must not beat or impede their intellect. On the contrary, the child must be given increasingly more encouragement. Let us assume that the child was able to do the swing by themself then the parent must have the ability to console them at the earliest and let them know that they did the job themselves. In this way, the child will transform themself into a guardian and eventually, will come to a decision that they can do things all by themselves. Though, if the parent rebukes and gives the child a harsh scolding then certainly, the child will not learn the nitty-gritty of learning and will clamor to yell and obscene issues. This the way that the child can actually transform their-self and get all the instincts risen through it.

The display of mutual work and integrity

Integrity comes with passion and mutual work. Montessori believed that if the child is allowed to learn in a multilateral manner then they can actually display a great sense of encouragement for the coming days of their life. For this principle to be followed, it's necessary that the classroom or the home be designed in an affectionate way. If you have two children or kids playing with you then you must be caring enough that you allow the child to grow progressively. The child must be given encouragement, so they finally get to achieve all the possible intellect of their-self. The modus operandi can be very easy and productive to understand. The children must applaud on working together. Make sure to not treat each other in an arch manner. They must be allowed to be given more momentum and relish when they see the works of mutuality. It all depends on parents how they want to see their child grow in their homes following the principle of Montessori.

Holistic Development of Students

Three types of developments manly affect the education of a child. The motor development, perceptual development, cognitive development, volitional development and emotional development are the developments that cater to the holistic upbringing of a child and without them a child can't progress in the society. The motor development is the development that defines the movement of a body and it's related to the neurotic messages that are sent from the brain to the body. How quick a child is able to respond to a stimulus of any environment is the motor development and such a development becomes very apparent in the contemporary era. The perceptual development defines the core perceptions of a child that how are they able to build their perception about anything in their life. In today's world, the perception from society to a state building narrative is very significant and without any opinion, the child isn't able to contribute to society. By contribution, it is not meant that a child becomes an astute politician. Although, the Montessori Method defines those necessary parameters that create a perception in a child's mind.

The thriving layers of Positivity through Montessori method

How can any problem or dilemma be finished from the cute minds of the toddlers? The answer is simply that they must be taught positivity and acceptability in the beginning of their lives. The aspect of positivity encourages toddlers to be more active, and they can get to the top of the food chain. For that, the teachers and parents must induce the feelings of love, passion, work and hard work in the minds of the toddlers. If they are able to do it then they have made strong and able children in the coming time. For this purpose, they can arrange some pictorial things in the class, they can tell some poems and proses that can give kids the notions of positivity. They can encourage kids of certain tendencies and elements in them due to which the toddlers will never feel alone and disconnected in their lives. There must be the independency of their choices and careers by the teachers and if the parents are teaching them at home, then the parents must also give them true powers. This prowess of independence is crucial to inculcate a layer of positivity in the minds of the children and every passing time, the children will get the portfolios of positivity in all ways necessary. Consequently, the indictment of positivity in the minds of the toddlers will yield great benefits for the children and then they will learn the harsh realities in a faster phase. This process needs to be taught and implemented by the parents in all layers of the class and home as well.

Individualism in a child

Montessori believed that children are habitual of making their own cognition. they would often observe children indulging in their own modes of creative art and they would deduce good educational results out of it. they believed that if children are to be given free platforms of learning, they can actually learn from it and can further, harness it, to the extreme level of success one can possibly imagine. For an instance, there is a class of twelve students, six students are given free discretions of choosing their educational modes of learning like they want teachers to sing for them and their own educational frameworks, given to them. On the contrary, the remaining six are taught in a traditional framework of education that is based on grueling learning and compelling memorizing. Under such circumstances, Montessori concluded that the first half of students will think more and create better things because they are not compelled to do things instead, they can perform their own abilities having their own discretion of it. In this way, a culture of individualism is present in a Montessori Method for teaching pupils and it can boost more individualism among the children.

Creation of well-structured routines

A Montessori routine will try its best to create discipline and love in the minds of the young toddlers. The major idea in this notion is the acceptability of discipline and amazement in the minds of the toddlers. Let us first understand what is meant by a well-structured routine. In the well-structured routine, the toddlers will know about academia, music and other beneficial hobbies. The first job is for the toddler is to get the intrinsic idea of learning. For that, this Montessori principle wants the toddler to learn all the things of academia before night and evening. Then when the evening has arrived, the toddler will be given an extra-curricular activity that they enjoy. They will be taught that how important it is to strive on a daily basis and they when they acquire this idea then they will work on it at the earliest. Why? Because this mere concept of a well-structured idea will increase the nourishment of the toddlers and in the coming time, they will meet the challenges of life. There are many impediments to it as well. The first hurdle is that the toddler might argue or forcibly try to avert the discipline of the well-structured routine. The second in line will be that the toddler will force you to come in their clout of innocence. The third can be any like trying to do something else. However, as long as you have over-shadowed your self-ego and have believed in the mechanism of the organization, then you do not have to worry about it because these steps and principles are designed to boost the mentality of the child by all ways possible. So, try your best in giving a confident boost to the toddlers at all means necessary. This is your responsibility to allow the working of this routine otherwise chaos and miseries will follow you in the forthcoming.

How liberty is accessed in the child's mind through the Montessori Methods

Do you want your child at home to come in cognition with the aspects, principles and assertions of Montessori school of thought at your home? Do you think that the school is doing a fine job in teaching the proper modes of liberty and independency through Montessori in you during the school days? If all the suspiciousness is true, then it's essential that the child might give you the green signal to teach and guide them about the libertine possibilities at home.

If you give your choice enough freedom and thought that they can actually be all the free lad that they yearn to be at home, then you are making them ready for the coming life. Let us suppose your child has shown some of the interests in becoming a doctor. Obviously, they won't say be their mind or face but in real terms, they will get all the possible help from their parent. A parent can draw a chart of a doctor and medical requirements to the child and let them know how the doctor works. By cute gestures and innocent use of tactics, the child can come in the cognition of all the myths of better understanding. The essential requirements for it are always in the hands of the parent that they must pictorially or visually help the students to inculcate a sense of glamor and help for the toddlers.

Just let the child know what they want at the moment and how will they able to transform their life in different ways. Do not be harsh on them and tell them what kind of virtues, a doctor possesses when they come to work. Show them the mode of working for the doctor, show them the dress-code of the doctor and by all means necessary, induce a successive mode of aspiration for them. These are the basic tenets of liberty that the child will first know independently that at what level they have to become a Montessori and how the tenure will work for them in the coming time. There is a grueling force of disturbance for the child in such a case, but it all makes sense, if the child has been able to understand the working of an individualistic profession at an early age.

Chapter 2: Toddler Mental Development

Mental development is a fundamental factor of increase, embracing the diverse mental skills. It starts proper from the beginning, and as the kid develops with time their intellectual reactions additionally change. Those reactions are quite simple initially, but in due path, they lead to complicated mental activities. Intellectual development includes such talents as attending, perceiving, observing, remembering, imagining, questioning, and solving troubles and growth of intelligence in addition to the language. These skills trade develop and mature with age and decline in old age. The quotes of alternate vary with age and special reviews. Notwithstanding a preferred pattern of intellectual improvement, each character grows and develops their own characteristic manner. The various intellectual skills or sports noted above are inter-associated and that they expand as an entire. They're inter-structured and do no longer increase in isolation. Except for this, 'inter-dependence, some other usual characteristic of mental improvement is its continuity. Intellectual development is another name for extending the highbrow horizon of the kid. To begin with, the sector is one big, "booming, humming confusion" to the child. Gradually, details are perceived and understood, variations are realized, and reviews and know-how are organized into new family members. This is made achievable through methods of differentiation and company or integration. The elements that affect intellectual improvement encompass maturation, learning and training. The type of fearful system the human infant inherits is an essential factor. It enables them to coordinate numerous sports and responses. It regulates the hobby of all the organs. The mind, a crucial part of the apprehensive device, plays a better sized role inside the mental development of the person than another component. It enables in the perception of the encircling world and notion is the idea of the mental activity – all idea and recognition.

Stages of Mental Development:

From Birth to Three Years:

The child is born with all the sensory gadgets which might be needed for mental pastime. With the aid of the age of 3, they portray the ability to satisfy their wishes selectively. Therein lays their mental improvement. This is obvious from different styles of behavior as well. they secure or tries to be relaxed

From Three to Six Years:

This period of the child's life is characterized by their capacity to apply symbols and phrases. They acquire a spread of sensory and perceptual experiences and these reviews contribute lots toward their mental development.

Later Childhood:

This era is marked with the aid of the potential to gather a keen and correct notion. With keen and correct belief grows the method of conceptualization. Mental improvement is also indicated in their growing interests. They start to evolve to respect matters and people around themself. They begin to mimic the manners and behavior of those humans whom they admire.

The Various Aspects of Mental Development:

Sensation and Perception:

Sensation and notion form an essential thing of intellectual improvement. The sensation is stepping one to understanding but it assumes the form of information best whilst it is attended to and a means is connected to it. In different phrases, sensations are objectified and end up meaningful. Objectified sensations are referred to as perceptions. To begin with, the surroundings of the child are an indistinct, undifferentiated mass attributable to the dearth of preceding experience and the undeveloped conditions of the feel organs. Gaining experience, the kid's sensations of taste, shade, sound, contact or stress get related to sure concrete gadgets. Gradually, the kid begins to see differences. They discriminate between matters and are aware of meanings. They also observe minute variations in quantities and members of the family; on the alternative they organize their know-how into new members of the family and "gestalts," in keeping with the gestalt college of psychology. However, it also entails memory pictures of the beyond revel in of the equal item or a comparable item. Our beyond reports which can be liable for the improvement of personal pursuits and intellectual sets are critical elements in belief. The child perceives those things quickly and really which can be concerned together with their interests and intellectual units. The kid's perceptions are also decided by way of their needs and goals. In a test, businesses of children – one, a bad group and the opposite a rich organization had been asked to perceive surely and choose the dimensions of the diverse coins shown to them. The terrible group overrated the dimensions of the cash extensively greater than did the rich group due to the fact to the terrible group, the cash were of notable cost and use.

Because the human man or woman grows older and enters early life or maturity, different factors that affect their perceptions are their ideals, opinions and cultural ideals. The sensations and perceptions are of 8 sorts. These are tactual, gustatory, olfactory, natural, kinesthetic, bodily equilibrium, auditory and visible, called so due to the experience organ involved – the skin, the tongue, the nostril, belly, muscle groups, semi-circular canals, the ear and the attention.

Concept Formation:

A concept is generalized which means this is attached to an item. It's a long way the result of our perceptual reports. As an example, 'horse' or 'house' or 'table' or 'honesty' or 'guy' are principles. We see several horses, homes or tables, see their commonplace features and traits and relations and finally arrive at a generalized perception. While we are saying horse, it was not this horse; it stands for all styles of horse. We hence arrive at concepts of factors, individuals and qualities, due to our perceptual enjoy, our ability to compare the commonplace traits, to narrate them to every different, to abstract and generalize. ‘residence’, ‘table’, ‘cap’ are standards of things; ‘father’, ‘mother’, ‘trainer’ are principles of humans, and ‘honesty’, ‘truthfulness’ are principles of traits and ideas. The formation and acquisition of ideas is a big breakthrough inside the mental development of kids. It entails both discrimination and generalization. The kid’s standards of the world increase with enjoy and together with their capability to understand relationships among new and old situations. Now not best do the ideas boom in number, with elevated rich and varied revel in, those principles end up richer and fuller. The ideas of December may have a specific implication if the kid has experienced it in Punjab, Delhi, Mumbai and Kolkata. It’s far away because of this that contemporary teaching secures the help of journeys, tour and visits to places of interest, for making their experiences richer and fuller. Such studies and contacts will surely deliver extra meaningfulness and breadth to the concepts shaped. Enjoying isn't the most effective component that contributes to comprehensiveness fashioned. Because when kids get older, they're in a position to examine extra books, magazines, ask questions from understanding human beings: in this way, they increase ideas of humans, matters and thoughts.

The concepts formed by the children in the early stages, are difficult to study for three reasons:

Many of the child’s concepts have meanings that might be unique from the ones of adults hence the grownup may overlook them. For a child, ‘doggie’ may also imply all small animals while to the adult, the concept of 'canine' is precise. The kid's standards are broad and more well-known rather than specific.

The kid's standards aren't formulated properly sufficient for the kid for you to express them in phrases comprehensible to a person.

Many children's standards cannot be 'verbalized' using them as a result of confined vocabulary.

Children's principles of spatial relations, of distance and intensity, are vague and inadequate in the beginning. That is chargeable for a great deal of the awkwardness in younger kids glaring at their miscalculations and distance language development focused on the know-how of the phrases like on, in, under, above, up and down, facilitates them to recognize spatial relations. The development of time takes vicinity, in starting the connection with wanting gratifications and being habitual. They recognize what morning and night suggest in phrases of feeding, eating and snoozing. Through the age of five, they may be capable to differentiate between the existing, past and destiny. How we degree time, they can recognize only with the aid of ten or so. Instructors of arithmetic want to understand those facts which might be results of investigations. The ideas of number and quantity are first added to the home to the minds of children by experiences within the domestic which bring to them the ideas of 'much less' or 'more' or 'being heavy' or 'mild'. Following the ideas of Jean Piaget, the Swiss Psychologist renowned for his research into the minds of children, kids gather principles of wide variety even earlier than they should and may be no longer capable of the count. They come in advance than the ones of weight. If domestic and school can offer concrete reports with a variety of substances, these concepts are discovered on time in a natural way. Medical ideas with subject causal relations expand whilst children are supplied with an expansion of troubles and they provide an explanation for or answer questions. Those concepts main to capacity in deductive and inductive reasoning develop with advancing age. Concepts of the self and social ideas of non-public relations greatly affect the child's questioning and behavior – a completely critical step within the intellectual improvement of children. To begin with the concept of self-approach simplest physical identity of self. Progressively, the child differentiates their-self from others. The child's social standards are encouraged via the character of inter private dating at home, with the aid of their reviews of others inside the neighborhood, within the playground and with the aid of other social sports. Also, the child develops concepts of beauty or aesthetic principles, through their contacts, their readings, institutions, cultural values, their experiences of coloration, Voice and form, i.e., environmental consequences. If the kid lives in dirty, drab and colorless surroundings there's a probability that they develop incorrect concepts of splendor of coloration, form or sound. Training and education and models in the house play a vital function in dedication of the nature of such ideas.

How to Improve Children's Mental Health?

As a parent, you frequently take your toddler to receive immunizations, provide healthy food to keep them healthy and examine plenty of books to develop their vocabulary. How regularly, do you think about how to attend to your infant's intellectual fitness? In case you're like many adults, it isn't that regular. But a toddler's intellectual fitness is just as crucial as them physical fitness, specifically in relation to conduct and academics. It's predicted that 1 in 5 children enjoy an intellectual disease in any given year, according to the centers for disorder management and prevention. And even as no longer all mental fitness troubles can be avoided, you may take steps to help maintain your baby as mentally healthful as achievable.

Pay Attention to Your Psychological Health

One of the best matters you may hold your toddler mentally wholesome to is to take care of your own mental fitness. No longer will you be modeling the behavior that improves mental health; though, you may additionally be growing more healthy surroundings on your child. Whilst the mother and father have untreated mental fitness issues, children are much more likely to develop psychological fitness problems. Kids are at a greater danger of developing intellectual contamination whilst both mother and father have mental health problems. A figure's untreated intellectual contamination may make family existence inconsistent or unpredictable. It may also influence a figure's potential to discipline the children and may stress a couple's courting. The ones things take a toll on a child's psychological properly-being. If you have an intellectual fitness problem, get remedy. Research shows whilst a figure gets remedy or medication to address the intellectual infection, kids' symbols and indicators improve.

Build Trust

A baby's relationship with a parent plays a large function in an infant's mental health. Growing a feeling of safety and security starts with constructing consider among figure and baby. This means making sure your baby meets both their bodily and emotional wishes. This includes taking care of them when they're hungry, thirsty, warm or bloodless, as well as when they're scared or unhappy. Stay committed to what you think and declares what you believe. Empty threats, damaged guarantees, and inconsistent care will make it difficult on your baby to accept as true with you.

Foster Healthy Relationships with Others

The connection a toddler has together with their father and mother is critical, but it's not the best dating that subjects. A mentally healthy toddler can have several relationships with relatives such as grandparents and cousins, as well as pals and associates. Even if you're the type of person that loves to spend your time alone with your toddler, deliver them the possibility to connect to other human beings. Take a nighttime off and permit your baby to have a sleepover with grandma or their cousins.

Be Reliable

The significance of being consistent can't be overstated. Toddlers crave predictable surroundings, and know-how of what interests them, what they're going to be spending time with, what consequences they come across if they ruin regulations and what privileges they'll receive for correct conduct. Whether you've moved to a new metropolis, or you're going with a divorce, chaos and massive adjustments may be tough for kids. It isn't unusual for them to withdraw, develop traumatic, or start appearing out while they're suffering to address their feelings. Establishing an ordinary, staying steady along with your subject practices and ensuring your baby is familiar with what's taking place in their everyday life.

Teach Your Child Healthy Ways to Manage Stress

Even as it's critical to shield your baby from stressful occasions the pleasant you could—trauma can make a contribution to mental health troubles—you may prevent your child from experiencing pressure. The pressure is a part of life. Disagreements with pals, being cut from a sports activities crew, and failed homework assignments are certain to show up at one time or every other. Provide your baby with the skills they need to cope with those situations. While one child may find comfort in writing a journal, another one may want to call a pal whilst he's vexed. So, proactively pick out the actions your child can take to preserve their strain tiers in check whilst they're handling difficult instances.

Establish Healthy Habits

A healthy weight-reduction plan, an excellent night's sleep, and plenty of exercises aren't simply properly for your infant's physical fitness—they may be essential for their mental fitness too. Train them to expand healthful conduct with a view to hold their frame and their mind in true form. There are many studies that indicate mindfulness and gratitude have a huge impact on mental fitness. So, you may additionally need to comprise these into your lives and with this method, you can improve the whole family's intellectual fitness.

Develop Self-Esteem

Supporting an infant broadens their self-respect, which can deliver a full-size boost to their intellectual health, is two-fold for a figure: first, you need to do your part in boosting your child's pride. Second, you should teach your baby how to broaden their personal vanity. Here are a few methods to help your infant broaden wholesome self-esteem:

Provide Possibilities for Independence.

Children feel better about themselves when they're capable of do things on their personal. So, whether you're coaching your baby how to get dressed otherwise you're showing them that you believe in them to make their own grilled cheese sandwich, kids feel exact about themself when they're able to show competence.

Help Your Baby Develop Wholesome Self-Speak.

When your infant says something like, "I'll never be good at math," it could be tempting to mention, "of course you will." Although, that won't assist them with increasing a healthier internal communicate. When your infant says bad things then correct them, ask questions like, "what do you want to do to get better?" Or "what's the evidence that this is true?" Assist your toddler to draw healthier conclusions.

Encourage Your Infant to Expand New Abilities.

Help your baby discover them talents and interests. Get them concerned in activities and inspire them to paintings tough to get better.

Be the Perfect Model.

A child who sees a parent continuously setting them down or doubting their self. They are likely to mimic that behavior. If you have shallowness inside, then take steps to enhance your understanding of people and things and better your mind so you may be an amazing position model for your baby.

Play Together

A healthy child—both physically and mentally—needs to play. Absolutely, adults need activity too! Make time for paintings, chores and other responsibilities with your toddler, which shows them that they're well worth your valuable time. When spending time with you child you will construct a closer relationship and overcome potential miscommunication errors and this will make your child try more to come closer to you and enjoy your presence.

Growth in Thinking and Problem Solving:

There is growth in questioning and fixing issues. This follows the formation of standards with the help of simple language and is a vital aspect of intellectual development. Thinking is a manner of handling feelings, perceptions or principles. This requires controlling signals instead of managing artifacts and circumstances in a system. It is assumed that wondering and hassle-solving are things that occur in later stages of human development. The child, consistent with this assumption, cannot assume or reason logically. Piaget said that there are tiers in kids' thinking. In his earlier experiments he discovered that up until the age of 7 or 8 a child tends to reason only in phrases of remote or precise instances, they are incapable of real argument and feel no want for logical justification; they have difficulties in making generalizations or deductions. Different research displays that, the children earlier than seven or eight additionally ought to reason about cause-and-effect relationships. Nonetheless, most of the thinkers are of the view that the highest kinds of thinking were no longer constantly viable in advance than 10 or eleven. It's true that children display development in areas of questioning as they grow older. The younger the kid, the more their thoughts tend to center on immediate occasions and problems as distinctive from more remote concerns. They deal without problems of the concrete and instead with the abstract.

Younger kids are more likely to advance in trial and errors. Once more, adults are probable to attain a conclusion or correct solution extra speedy and to peer factors extra easily. Facing and solving problems is a crucial constituent of mental development. The preceding paragraph indicates that easy problem-fixing isn't always past the intellectual capacity of young kids. Even a child at the age of 3 makes an effort to remedy a tough scenario. Indeed, the hassle of the state of affairs regularly is private and concrete and their effort is typically marked through trial-and-error. Using insight, however, isn't always totally ruled out even within the initial years. To understand the abilities of young kids, adults need to perceive each problem and their answers from the child's point of view. If they examine it in terms of the common sense of a rational adult, they'll get an inaccurate view of a baby's conscience. "Kids can also have a terrific sensible draw close of the concept of the purpose-and-impact of their sphere of sports even though they cannot phrase the idea in logical terms."

The Growth of Intelligence or Intellectual Development:

Development or growth of intelligence is a crucial aspect of mental development. We will delineate such development now.

The growth of intelligence does not take relaxation away from the child's mind. Language improvement, emotional and social progress in addition to the physical growth is related to holistic development or the increase of intelligence. Over the past fifty years, many attempts have been made to research intelligence and its progress from start to maturity with the help of developmental faculties designed by Arnold Gessel, infant exams designed with the aid of Cattell, Stanford, Binet scale, Army Alpha, Otis' scale and Wechsler's checks for kids and adults, and many others on international grounds. With the help of those assessments, we're in a position to provide test for every age and may constitute them on a curve. Those scores have enabled psychologists to screen out children with extraordinary intelligence, to split the slow form the borderline cases, the advanced from the average group. We can observe the standard intellectual curve or the curve of intelligence that displays that infancy is marked with fast intellectual increase; is moderate then and it slows down in older kids. A few studies show that rankings stay steady or grow slowly in person lifestyles tend to say no in vintage age. Although, this is only true of a few components of intelligence. Different people have given exclusive types of curves, but all agree that intelligence will increase with age in an ordinary population. Of course, there are variations. Some individuals display a fast growth in fields of intelligence, whereas others show rapid growth in other regions. Those curves also point out intervals where there seems to be no rise i.e., durations of no progress, technically referred to as plateaus.

Checking the intelligence of a character over years, suggests the pattern of their growth. It also shows how steady their IQ is. The IQ or the ratio of the intellectual rise isn't regular in any inflexible experience, but what the repeated annual assessment suggests is that advanced kids remain superior and inferior kids continue to be inferior. After 6 years, there's greater fidelity of IQ. Then in later years. If there are any big fluctuations inside then by observing the scores over time, you see that these are due to factors such as fitness, interest or motivation, fatigue or, the sudden environmental changes or personal defects. Intelligence seems to grow on to a positive age that's its limit. Other elements of the mental progress are related to a child's memory, and creativeness. In this paragraph, we will talk in short about the memory and ability to remember for a child and how it progresses with intellectual rise. The developmental studies of reminiscence as discussed by Hurlock and Schwartz, suggest that the child, in the first 1/2 of the year, has reminiscence of an impressionistic kind. Proper remembrance solidifies at the end of the first year. Memories are created using sensory stimuli, to begin with, but by way of giving up of the second one 12 months, the kid is capable of considering ideas with the help of words or symbols. During the primary and 2nd years, toddler's reminiscence is more potent for people and objects than for conditions. Situations find a place in the toddler's memory at 3 to 6 years of age. The kid's memory is encouraged favorably or adversely with the aid of the emotions, find studies. It may be easier to remember extraordinary circumstances than unpleasant ones. Emotional improvement, the emergence of joy, expression and understanding of feelings start to grow during early life. The improvement of feelings takes place along with cognitive and behavioral improvement and emerges within a selected social and cultural context.

Chapter 3: Physical Developments of a Toddler

Sadly, for those parents that wish for their baby to stay innocent forever, life does not happen to work in their favor. Our babies rapidly grow into mini versions of us, and this means an entirely different phase is in store for naïve parents. Once the walking and talking begins, there is no turning back. The role of parenting comes to a whole new level which means your life and home will never be quite the same again.

Toddler Developmental Milestones

12 Months

They can utilize their feet to push themselves along on ride-on toys

They show interest in balls and playing with them.

At this age, throwing or tossing the ball to your child is key for some motor development. Begin by rolling a soft, small ball back and forth between you and your toddler, ensuring that you're gradually moving farther away. In time, they will eventually have the desire to throw it.

When teaching them to kick a ball, show them to use their feet instead of their hands.

To catch a ball, have them roll it up an incline to catch on the way down.

15 Months

They can walk without your help, but with the assistance of walking with their feet spread apart and their arms to contribute to proper balance

They can get themselves up from the sitting to standing positions by utilizing their hands to push themselves up and sit down with the use of their hands

They can bend down to pick things up themselves.

In time, this action will evolve to squat. To assist your toddler in developing this motor skill, when they start to bend over an object, show them how to bend their knees.

Practice makes perfect of course! Line up some toys and have them pick them up. This will also help in mental development of when clean-up time is as well.

18 Months

They can drink from a cup without assistance.

They can draw/scribble/write on paper using a variety of utensils.

They are capable of climbing onto low furniture.

Toddlers are inevitably going to attempt to climb whatever they think they can get on, because of the mere fact it is there.

Climbing is a vital physical development. So do not prohibit them from climbing, but rather create safe opportunities for them to do so. Throw sofa cushions on the floor and create a padded playground for them to enjoy.

Ensure that heavy furniture and other objects in your household such as bookcases and televisions are properly anchored down so that your child doesn't knock them over on themselves.

They can build a tower out of block-like toys.

They can now pick up small objects since they have practiced the pincer grip.

They are able to push wheeled toys in front of them.

Once your child becomes more confident in their walking abilities, they will desire pushing and pulling toys and other objects around. Ensure that during this stage, you offer them push or pull toys to play with.

2 Years

They have the ability to push buttons and turn knobs.

Most can walk down the stairs by holding onto the railing and placing both feet onto a step.

They can easily run in one direction and stop when they need to.

They are able to walk backwards.

They are capable of running.

Each child is different, but some toddlers may go from crawling to being able to sprint at rapid rates in what seems like a matter of seconds. Some children take risks faster than others.

Encourage your toddler to play tag on softer areas, such as sand or grass.

Chase your child around, encouraging them to run from you. Then have them chase you around.

They are capable of getting themselves off the floor without using their hands.

They can take off articles of clothing.

2 ½ Years

They can undress themselves.

They are learning the ways to pick out clothes and dress themselves properly.

They can throw a large ball in the direction they intend.

They can walk upstairs.

They can kick a large ball, even though it usually does not go in the direction they intend to.

They can feed themselves with the utilization of a spoon.

They can drink from a normal cup.

They can get on and off playground equipment.

They can run smoothly (and with speed).

3 Years

They can feed themselves using both a spoon and a fork.

They have begun the potty-training process.

This is the milestone that parents look forward to maybe the most because this means no more diapers! The age at which your toddler can properly go to the washroom can vary greatly. Here are signs that your toddler may be ready to start the process of potty-training:

Looks down at diapers and grabs or pulls them off when soiled.

Crosses their legs or squats when they need to go.

Shows interest in potty-related things, such as discussing pee or poo or wants to watch you go to the bathroom.

They are capable of throwing and catching a ball if they utilize two hands.

They can kick a ball with more force.

They have the capability to jump.

Toddlers during this stage will begin to jump off the ground or off low objects. Jumping requires bilateral coordination skills as well as the ability to utilize both sides of the body.

Encourage "curb hopping". Hold your toddler's hand and stand next to a curb or step and say "One, two, three… jump!" then jump down with them.

Teach them to leapfrog. Demonstrate how to get down into a half-squatting position and to throw their arms up in the air while hopping.

They can balance themselves and are able to walk on tippy toes.

They can walk both up and down the stairs without the parent's help.

They can begin to play with ride-on toys like bicycles.

The toddler stage is quite a unique one during human development, in fact, toddlers are no longer considered babies, but they are not considered to be preschoolers either. There are a lot of crucial developmental components that occur during this timeframe, which is why as parents we should always be encouraging growth and watching for signs that show our young child may be falling behind developmentally. Of course, all children learn and grow at different paces.

Gross Motor Development

Gross motor skills are physical capabilities that utilize large bodily movements that require the entire body. During the time, your child is a toddler, they stop toddling and look particularly awkward when they walk. They begin to walk and can do so more smoothly. They are able to run and at much faster rates, as well as hop and jump. They have the capability to actively participate in throwing and catching a ball and can push themselves around by themselves or while upon a riding toy.

Fine Motor Development

Fine motor movements are vastly different than gross motor skills, since they require the ability to utilize precise movements to adequately perform. During the toddler stage, children can begin to create things with imagination by their own hands. They can create towers out of toy blocks, mold clay into recognizable shapes, and are more than capable of scribbling on paper with crayons or pens. They quite enjoy toys that allow them to insert specific shapes into one another. This is also the time parents will start to notice which hand their child prefers to use over the other, as they begin to become either right-handed or left-handed.

Signs of Developmental Issues

Like mentioned before, children learn and develop at different rates, so don't be too concerned if they aren't acquiring new skills at the same rate as a friend's or neighbor's kids. If you're concerned, it is best to talk to a health professional to clear up any concerns for the following reasons:

Ages 1–2 Years

If they aren't picking up small objects or unable to utilize a pincer grip.

If they are unable to hold up a spoon strong enough to feed themselves.

If they aren't walking at a steady pace or if they display a limp in their stride.

If they aren't walking at all yet.

Ages 2–3 Years

If they are totally unable to feed themselves with use of a spoon.

If they are not as active as their peers or siblings.

If they are not capable of walking upstairs or climbing low furniture.

If they do not have the ability to run smoothly.

Physical Appearances of a Toddler

By the end of their first 12 months here on planet earth, your 1-year-old's growth will predominantly be just their height and weight, as their next big growth spurt will not come again until the time of adolescence. Continue to write down their measurements each month to ensure your toddler is indeed still growing at the rate they should be.

At around 15 months, the average girl weighs around 23 pounds and is about 30.5 inches in height, while the average boy is 24.5 pounds and is around 31 inches tall. Over the course of a few months, they will probably only gain a pound or so and grow an inch at most. When your child reaches the "terrible two" stage, girls should weigh about 27 pounds and stand 34 inches tall, while boys will stand about 34.5 inches tall and weigh around 28 pounds. The circumference of their skull will probably only expand to another inch or so during this time. Around the age of 2 years, your child will have obtained 90% of the adult head size.

As for bodily appearance, that of a toddler will change more dramatically than their size will. At the age of 12 months, your child still has a baby-like appearance, with their abdomen and head being the largest part of their bodies. As they start to become more active, they will develop core muscle strength, which will aid in shedding some of that precious baby fat. Legs and arms will lengthen over time, and their feet will point in the direction they are walking. Their faces will start to have a more angular appearance, with a better-defined jaw line. It will be rather difficult to recall what your child looked like as an infant by the time they are 2 years, so remember to take plenty of photos before this time!

Even though there aren't as many dramatic or noticeable changes as to your child's physical appearance during the time they are 2–3 years old, they will continue to make grand strides in development as they transform from a mere baby to an active child. Probably the most dramatic occurrences during this time are their bodily proportions. As an infant, your child's head was quite large, and they had pretty short arms and legs. During the toddler stage, the head will grow much less as the arms and legs play catch-up, with the rest of their bodies. Different portions of their body will begin to look much more proportional. All that baby fat that once made your baby so darn cuddly will slowly begin to fall off, especially during the pre-school years. Arms and legs will become much thinner as will their faces. Their posture will become less pudgy like as their once protruding abdomens and curving lower back start to extend to an upright position. This is thanks to their drastic increase in muscle tone, which can assist in keeping their bodies at a much more human-like stance.

Do not become too worried if your toddler eats less than you think they ought to be by the time they turn 2 years of age. Children during this time in their life need fewer calories to burn because they are growing at a slower rate. Ensure that you're providing your child a healthy array of foods, especially during this time. This will aid in proper mental development, as explained in the following chapter. This is a great time as any to encourage good eating habits. Ensure that your child does not seem too preoccupied with food or gains excessive amounts of weight because this could be a sign of an undiagnosed condition or could influence bad eating habits later in life.

Chapter 4: Applying the Montessori Method at Home

The Montessori method was developed over 100 years ago by Maria Montessori. This method of learning focuses on the belief that all children have the capacity to independently initiate their learning experiences. Montessori schools and classrooms contain a compelling combination of activities and materials which are specifically designed to develop learners who are well rounded. This means that the children who learn through the Montessori method are challenged emotionally, socially, physically, and cognitively.

Montessori isn't an unknown term in the world of education. Even though parents may not know what Montessori all is about, they must have already heard of it. One of the best things about Montessori is that children can learn through this method even in the comfort of their own home. From the Introduction of this book all the way to Chapter 5, you have learned a lot about Montessori.

When it comes to applying the Montessori method and its principles at home, there are some things you must do. Now that you've learned more about the different areas of Montessori, you have a better idea of the types of materials and activities you can create (or purchase) for your child. But the Montessori method isn't just about that. Before we end our discussion, here are some final tips to guide you:

Prepare the environment

When it comes to the prepared environment of Montessori, keep in mind that there's always a proper place for everything. Assign one of the rooms in your home as your child's Montessori learning environment. If there are Montessori schools in your area, go ahead and visit them to have a better idea of how to arrange this room.

You may also go online and search for Montessori classroom ideas on Google or Pinterest. Either way, having a visual image of what Montessori classrooms must look like will give you a better idea of how to arrange the room you've assigned in your own home. One thing to keep in mind though is to make sure that everything is child-sized and at your child's level so that they won't keep asking you for assistance when they need something.

Plan all the materials and activities to include in your child's environment

After planning the environment, it's time to think about the materials to place and activities to establish inside that environment. You can go online to search for a complete list of Montessori materials in each of the learning areas. Then you can either purchase similar materials (actual Montessori materials are very expensive) or create them on your own. For instance, you can easily create sandpaper letters and numbers using thick cardboard and sandpaper.

Arrange these materials and activities according to their areas of learning and make sure that all of them are accessible to your child. You may want to include a combination of easy materials and those which are a bit more challenging or unfamiliar to your child. Also, you may want to rotate these items regularly, so your child doesn't get bored. If you see that he's not interested in some activities or they have already mastered others and they're not using them anymore, take these materials out and replace them with new ones.

Focus on life skills

Children should learn life skills early on. With these skills, children learn how to care for themselves and their environment. This sets children up to become capable and considerate adults when they grow up. Providing the proper materials to teach these skills even makes your life as a parent a lot easier! Soon, your child will start volunteering to help you around the house because they already know how to do these chores.

Of course, you must always match the activities and materials to the abilities and age of your child. Introducing activities which are too difficult for children is never a good idea. Obviously, your child won't be able to do these activities and if you force him, this might weaken their self-confidence and their willingness to continue with the rest of the activities you've prepared.

Help your child learn concentration and inner motivation

These skills are essential if you want your child to get the most out of the Montessori method. For a child to master a skill, concept or activity, they must concentrate while doing it. If you have prepared the environment well, your child will be able to concentrate on the activities you have prepared for them. This means that there should be no distractions such as gadgets, electronic devices, and random toys which don't really have a purpose inside the room.

Also, avoid giving your child rewards when they do something good or gain proficiency in something. Try to observe your child when they realize that they have finally been able to master a puzzle or a practical activity. You will see a sense of accomplishment in your child. This is much more valuable than extrinsic rewards because this sense of accomplishment becomes the driving force within your child to keep on going in order to master the other activities in their environment.

Take on the role of a Montessori teacher

Finally, learning how to facilitate the Montessori method for your child is also essential. Rather than teaching everything to your child, allow them to discover, explore, and choose the materials and activities on their own. If your child asks for help, oblige. If not, observe.

You may also step in if your child picks up a material and can't figure out how to use it. Again, they will probably ask you to help them out. These are the best and most appropriate times to step in when it comes to the Montessori method. Then when your child celebrates their mastery of a skill, celebrate with them! There's nothing more satisfying than to see your child grow, develop, and improve at their own pace and through their own efforts.

Montessori is truly a wonderful learning approach. Whether it's done in school or at home, children love learning through this method mainly because of how it's done. Now that you've learned all the basics about Montessori, you may start planning how you'll apply this in your home. Then step back and watch your child learn it the ideal way!

Chapter 5: Teach Cooperation

Cooperation can yield many prospects for the growth of the child, but it requires a lot of hard work and skill. You're cooperating with the child, who is just a toddler and needs your affectionate companionship at all cost. You cannot be robust neither you can induce horrific compulsions among them. But you must nourish the fundamentals of care and start by listening to them. You can observe their notions and you can stay connected with their memories at a longer run. However, the question arises that what can be the potential methods of inducing cooperation in the children? Well, the answer is as follows:

Ways to be cooperative with the kids

Following are the ways to be cooperative with your kids

Taking turns

While we are taking turns, we are boosting team management and cooperation among the toddlers. We need to understand that the baby is all growing up and they are imitating the notions of all the elders in a respected manner. They need to understand that while growing up, the life pattern can be very dangerous and the one, who can cooperative and compassionate, can only yearn to be successful. An example can be portrayed here to understand the thinking of the child. While they are playing blocks and or creating a puzzle, let them do their modes alternatively. You should take turns while you're building blocks for them and then you have to see, what they do in return. So, taking turns means that you have to be a team player and you have to be cooperative with them at all cost.

Explain your reasons for limits and reasons

A controlled environment is very pertinent to reflect good progress in society. It is the only way through which success and sustainability can be achieved in the team. You need to explain to the child that they are the only benefactor of this process and you have to make sure that they follow all the rules of the house. In this way, the house will be in order and they will perceive management and order in a perpetual way. Hence, this model of cooperation, can be very effective for the soul and heart of the child and you need to induce this method in all ways necessary.

Take time to problem solve

You should take time to see if the kids are capable of solving the dilemmas that come in their life. Problems like the breaking of a glass, the absence of any material and the overall loss of any prodigal thing can be termed as examples. Thus, when such dilemmas appear, the parent must ask many minutes and good questions to the child. Like what seems to be the problem baby, how can the problem be solved, is there any potential solution to it? If so, then what is the alternative to it. When the child finds answers and if the answers are polite and keen, then please do encourage. This encouragement will give cooperative clout to the children and hence, the child will be able to yield more love for the parent.

Do chores together start at an early age!

You need to mentally encourage your child to do chores with you. This means that if you're washing the dishes then you must allow your child to share the burden of work with you. If you're washing your car then you must bring your child into the work as well. Moreover, any burden of a work, which is being conducted and shared by you, must be allowed to be executed by your child as well. In this way, the child will learn how to cooperate with the parent and will come one step closer to the field of house-living. If you do not do it and do not allow the child to host, you; properly then you will see negative results of their upbringing. Therefore, it is necessary that you see your child get the very best of housework and do all your best in making the child look cleaner and more efficient.

Giving more praise for cooperative efforts

If your child is doing something cooperative, then do please them and give them thumbs up. Otherwise, they won't reconcile with you. The child can do a lot of work once they is given a boost and some mental encouragement. They can thaw their weaknesses and can convert it into happiness. They can see the role of their efforts in a progressive manner and can make the uttermost of the house routine. If you see the cooperation of others, then please do let your child learn the art of cooperation as well. Also, giving them more praise will clear all the mental barriers in their head about parenting and they will come one step near you in many aspects. Thus, more praise can lead your child to the cooperation they deserve.

Always be suggestive

Never be compulsive or orderly to your children. Always look to it that they have a caring parent that is suggesting them to do more and more things. If you find a mistake in them then do correct them genuinely and never let other things come in the way. Once you do bad things for the child, you will ultimately be surrounded with issues. Your child will become paranoid and you'll make a mess of your life. Therefore, suggestions to your child will always lead to more innocence and cooperation in the child.

Give your child choices while maintaining the rules

You are maintaining the order in your child but at the same time you want them to be cooperative. So, under such circumstance, it is very pertinent that you're suggestive to all the actions of your child and let the child be on the same path with you. For instance, before bed, if you want your child to be following the rules then ask them politely if they have brushed their teeth and are their diapers clean. These cute and innocent questions will liberate the child from tension, and they will cooperate more.

Talk your child about their feelings and let them know yours

Talk to your child about the feelings they have and let them know the prospects of it as well. Let them see how they can communicate it with you and how you will transform yourself within the limits. The child is able to harness more potential in this sense and will tell you about their progress in any field. They will come to know about the possibilities of life and will be very close to you in any regard. Hence, always be communicative with your child and never allow any emotional disturbance to impede your affiliation.

Explain them the situations in a calm manner

Explain to them the reasons why sad expectations come in the way. And do not yell at them while you're doing so. If by chance, they are not able to clear any exam then it isn't your obligation to defame them. Just be a kind parent and let them understand the possibilities of life in an affectionate manner. Try to suggest them more cooperative tactics that will enable them to yearn enjoyment. So, the explanation of tough situations in an easy way that will make your child more cooperative and substantial.

Play games with them

Games like cricket and football are very effective to boost creativity and subjectivity in the kids. If you hold a bat and hit your child's ball, the child will learn cooperation by all means necessary. Even if you're playing the game of football with them and you're running alongside them and telling them how to kick; then you are being cooperative, and the child will be more productive to your advice and to learning. Therefore, play as much of the games, you want to play with them and in the end, you'll end up being very affectionate with them. This is one of the most effective and splendid methods in making the child know the cooperation platform and you should feel proud if you're doing so.

Always ask permissions before joining

Always ask permissions to your child if you're about to join them and see what the child can do. If your child is playing the match of cricket and you're watching them then try your best in not disturbing them, if you're washing the dishes and the child is watching movies then ask their permission to join them. These examples assert your cooperative and affectionate behavior with the child and eventually, lead the child to a better end. But if you are arrogant and stubborn enough to vociferously scold them then you must not expect any kind of cooperation from the child. Because the child will be very stubborn for you and they won't learn the art of cooperation.

Sharing is caring

If you're a busy guy and have a tough schedule on your time, then try your best in complying with your child. It is understandable that the child will not get your routine and with innocent questions and jolly mood, everybody can calm down. For instance, the child can get to the bottom of your routine and you're having a tough time dealing with them so in such a circumstance, you must adhere to all the disciplinary steps that can navigate obedience in your child and hence, you need to share things with him, in order to achieve cooperation from their side. Hence, they will care for you if you share your routine with them.

So, with such ways and measures, the term cooperation can be easily put forward to the students and children as well.

Chapter 6: Kind-Minded Parenting

Mental parenting is an approach that recognizes children's independent thoughts and feelings. Parents assume that the actions of their children are significant and respond to the feelings, preferences, and expectations of their children. We interpret the communicative signals of their children correctly and talk to kids about the mind world.

The approach is linked to significant developmental advantages, such as forging secure attachment relationships, strengthening social skills, and possibly improving self-control.

Some of the behavioral differences that we see within families illustrate genetic differences. Our genes will give us a greater or lesser chance of developing those skills.

But there is good evidence that matters relating to parenting and caregiving, and this is especially true for stable relationships and mind skills theory.

Kind-minded parenting tuning in and making thoughtful mental state observations strengthen social bonds and help children understand other people's thoughts and feelings. Hence, there is reason to think that focused parenting will help children to develop better self-control.

Montessori at Home and Montessori Parenting

The parenting of Montessori is a big part of the Montessori philosophy. To raising a Montessori child bridging the gap between school and home is key. Consult with the teachers in your child to make this happen.

Life offers children moments of encouragement. Let them put the shoes on themselves. Offer support for them without doing so. Don't take for granted that you have the solution or can solve their problem. Children can do a lot. Respecting our children's potential for growth and development based on their impulses and preferences is just as much a part of the Montessori classroom as it is part of the Montessori home environment.

Opening our eyes to that possibility is crucial to Montessori integration at home. The universe is our classroom at the risk of sounding out cliché. What Dr. Montessori stressed included an approach to engaging with children, disciplining children, directing children, and preparing the atmosphere to ensure a child's development is successful.

Toddlers Communication

The desire for independence: In order to become a responsible adult, your child must move slowly from the passenger seat to the driver's seat and learn to drive the tortuous paths of life.

For children, everything is black or white for example, for a child, the concept of justice is simple: 'Mama broke a cookie and gave half to me, half to my brother.' In this case, justice comes down to a mathematical formula. Abstract thinking helps your child draw their or them own conclusions about complex issues. But this has a downside: their conclusions may be contrary to yours.

What You Can Do

Have relaxed conversations. Enjoy the moments when your child is more comfortable to talk. Be brief. You do not need to give a long sermon to every problem. Say what needs to be said and stop there. This may take effect later. When your child is alone, they will be able to think better about what you said. Give them a chance to do it.

Listen and be flexible. To get a full picture of the problem, listen carefully - without interrupting. When you say something, be reasonable. If you stick to the rules too much, your child will be tempted to look for loopholes. That's where the children begin to lead a double life. They tell parents what parents want to hear, but they do what they like when they are away from them.

Always give guidance instead of orders unless you really have to. Your child's ability to think abstractly is like a muscle that needs to be exercised. So, when they need to make a decision, do not do the "exercise" for them. When discussing the problem, let them suggest some solutions. Then say something like, "Now that you have given some options think of them for a day or two. Then we can talk about which one you prefer and why".

Starting from the point that parents are the best friends of children and they just want to see their happiness and satisfaction, why not be the best medium of information for them? And be able to help them?

There are many factors that cause a lack of intimacy between parents and their children, making it difficult for the family to communicate:

- Lack of meetings during meals

- Parents work late and hardly see their children

- At weekends, kids prefer television, video games or the internet than sit down for a family conversation

- When they are with their parents, children do not reveal their problems because they feel ashamed, the contact is so little that sometimes it is better to talk with a friend in the school with whom they interact daily than to talk with the father and mother who only finds them at night and seldom.

It's hard to really communicate with someone you do not know well. Do you know your child? Children need to feel that adults trust them. Many, given the opportunity, will be worthy of the trust deposited in them. And it is very good for parents to be able to speak openly and honestly about their own youth, as they did then. It shows a high degree of confidence. Young people who can communicate with their parents are much happier and more confident. Sincere communication is the number one priority for young people. Efficient communication is based on:

- Having mutual trust.
- Show frankness and honesty.
- Be able to forgive and go forward.
- Respect privacy.
- Avoid joking and scorn.
- Maintain good humor and willingness to make real compliments
- Leave there the usual problems.
- Be able to listen and then talk.
- Move away and choose a better time when you're angry.
- Do not make accusations.

Showing interest in the children's lives is proving that parents care about them. Do you know the answers to these questions?

What is the name of your child's best friends? Have you been introduced to them yet? Do you know where they live? What kind of book, movie, and sport does your child enjoy? What is their team? What kind of music does they like? Do you know if you have any special subject, any area or hobby your child is interested in? If they practice a sport, do you know what position they play on the team? When was the last time you went to see them play?

It is extremely important to fraternal friendship. Children need their parents more than ever, the world each day is complicated in a frightening way, several problems afflict young people, and that is why the family needs to see the lack of communication and a more intimate relationship. All major modern things, such as TV, the Internet, and advertising, contributed to the family changing their habits, greatly facilitating the lives of individuals. The truth is that there is a lack of interest by the parents in the universe of the children and vice-versa, but this has a solution, it is enough to want and to be involved.

Speak Positively, But Praise the Effort More Than the Child

They also hear less praise. And since these children tend to listen to fewer words in general, these negative expressions end up having a greater weight in their cognitive development. What will it be like repeatedly to hear that you never do anything right? It's a difficult child environment to overcome. The difference between prohibition words ('do not do it,' 'stop') and encouragement ('very well') is great. It causes stress in the brain to hear them repeatedly. It is necessary to try to change orders for a more productive conversation.

But if negative and prohibitive language can be a barrier to development and learning, is the answer always to praise - and constantly say that your child is incredible and intelligent?

Chapter 7: Art and craft activities

The Montessori activities on art and craft can teach a thing or two about organization and order. Toddlers' materials for these activities should be easy to get to, well organized, striking, suitable for their age, appealing, and guileless. The most useful aspect of art and craft material for toddlers is their simplicity. The materials are expected to enhance creativity, hone fine motor abilities and improve coordination and sharp focus.

For these activities, it is essential to avoid the compilation of clutter and waste. The following steps should guide parents and teachers when teaching art and craft activities.

Use a few materials. Toddlers need to be presented with few materials at a time. The fewer materials presented to the toddler the fewer the chances of wasting and mess.

Present a manageable number of activities. Do not overwork the toddler with loads of activities. There still is time for the toddler to master the concepts. Rotate the activities frequently but don't engage the toddler with many activities at the same time.

Use baskets and trays. Always provide the art and craft materials in a basket or a tray. The containers help in making the materials easy to get to and keep the materials safe and orderly. The only exemptions would be water or paints.

Make the materials suitable for the age of the toddler. Suitability, in this aspect, means material that isn't dangerous to the health of the toddler. Do not use toxic materials or very complicated materials.

Present materials that encourage clean-up. Provide sponges, wet wipes, mops, etc. to allow the toddler to learn some cleaning after exercising the art activities. Small bins are very useful for discarding paper wastes.

With all this in mind now, let us take a look at a host of art and craft activities for your toddlers.

Drawing

Materials

For this activity, you need to present some color pencils in a box with a sliding lid, a paper, or canvas surface. Take note to rotate the color selection from time to time depending on the type of paper or surface you are using.

Step by step

Show the toddlers how to use their color pencils or crayons by drawing some simple patterns on the paper or canvas material.

Let the toddlers take turns in drawing the patterns you have just showed them.

Remember to guide the toddlers step by step to inspire them to explore more, without being rigid, which may hinder their imagination.

Watercolor painting

Materials

Provide watercolors, brushes, a jar of water, and a plain surface (paper or canvas), and a pallet for mixing colors.

Step by step

Smear the desired color on a pallet.

Wet the bristles of the brush in water provided in a jar.

Mix the color on the pallet using the wet brush.

Paint some patterns on your flat surface.

Keep a piece of cloth to help in cleaning the area of exercise.

Cutting

Materials

Sturdy cards and a pair of scissors.

For this activity, teach the toddlers how to hold the scissor by the handle and remind them that the blades are sharp. The activity is recommended for age group 3 and above.

Step by step

Hold a piece of sturdy card on one hand and a scissor on the other.

Cut a thin strip off the card.

For younger kids, hold the paper for them as they use their two hands to hold the scissors and cut.

As the kids advance, start creating straight lines on the paper and cut along the lines. Let them repeat the process on their own.

Sewing

Materials

For this activity, you're required to provide sewing cards, cross-stitch needles

In a case and sewing threads.

Step by step

Hold the sewing card while showing the toddlers the holes in the card.

Show the toddlers how to sew the holes and rotate the card after each hole.

At this stage, let the toddlers pull the sewing thread through the holes and push the stitching needle through the next hole on the sewing card.

Cut the thread at the end and let them learn how to make a knot at the end of the thread.

Prick work

This activity is aimed at helping the toddlers learn how to control the movement of their hands.

Materials

A piece of paper, pricking object.

Step by step

Make patterns on the piece of paper. Start with simple patterns as you advance to complex drawings.

Let the toddlers prick holes along the patterns.

If possible, show the toddlers how to make holes all along with the shapes you have drawn. Help them pull out the shapes.

Punches

Provide paper punches on varied shapes and sizes like hearts, diamonds, or Christmas tree. Let the toddlers punch a piece of paper that you have provided and pull out the shapes made. This art activity helps them develop creative skills and make them learn about different shapes.

Gluing

Materials

Provide different shapes of paper images in a bowl, a small pot of glue and a brush. A separate flat paper is also required.

Step by step

Spread the sheet of paper on a flat surface, preferably a tabletop.

Using the brush with the bristles immersed in the pot of glue, spread the glue on the back of the shapes and images provided.

Slowly spread the shapes on the flat sheet of paper.

Let the toddlers try doing this on their own.

Modeling clay

This activity should involve toddlers in making different shapes using clay.

Materials

The supervisor should provide some modeling clay, a rolling pin, and some cookie cutters. Also, remember to provide a wet towel for cleaning once the activity is complete.

Step by step

Guide the toddlers in modeling different shapes using clay.

For flat shapes, place some clay on a flat surface and flatten the clay using the rolling pin.

Using the cookie cutter, cut the clay into different shapes.

Guide the toddlers in repeating the process.

As an alternative to the modeling clay, you also use colored playdough or kinetic sand.

Color Collage

This activity involves sticking different colored papers into matching colors on the flyer provided. Creating color collages helps develop creativity in toddlers.

Materials

Colored construction paper, bowls, flyers, scissors, and glue.

Step by step.

Cut the colored paper according to the color arrangement. Put different colors in separate bowls.

Pick one bowl containing cut pieces of paper of the same color. Read out the color to the toddlers and ask them to identify the color in the flyer you have provided.

Using the gluing skill, you had taught earlier, let the toddlers stick the pieces on the flyer with matching colors.

Making a color booklet

Materials

A sketchpad, labeled colored papers, glue, and crayons.

Step by step

Cut the labeled colored papers into one shape, preferably rectangle.

On the sketchpad, label every page with a different color on the top part of the page.

Let the toddlers identify the colored papers and help them stick every paper on the matching page of the sketchpad.

Leave a small margin on every page for the toddlers to paint the matching color using their crayons.

Handprint fall tree craft

This activity requires you to provide some bottles of paints and cotton swabs. Trace the outline of a tree on a piece of paper and let the toddler finish the leaves by dipping them fingers in paint and leaving their prints on the image. Random prints can give the image a very appealing look. The cotton swabs are used to clean the fingers to change to another color. After the activity, have your toddler wash them hands.

Paper shape collage

If your toddler can draw, ask them to draw a random shape, say a triangle. Now have them introduce another shape in the triangle, say a circle. Tear colored papers of different colors and have your kid glue them to the image. Note that every shape should be given a different color of paper.

Creating Paper plate animals

Your toddler can make paper plates by finger-painting them. To create the paper plate animals, guide them in fixing paper faces and limbs. The activity offers the environment for nurturing creativity and awareness of the surrounding.

Sticker word activity

This is among the simplest art and crafts activities for the toddler. Have them write their name on a manila paper (offer help if they cannot write on their own). Offer the toddler a set of colored stickers to put on the name or word written. The stickers are put along the lines of the letters.

Colored straw necklace

For creative and elegance have your toddler exercise this activity. Provide colored straws. Help them cut the straws using a pair of scissors to the desired size. The sizes may vary. Using the threading technique, you have taught, let the toddler thread the straws together, and alternating the colors to give the necklace a beautiful look. For more designs, you can tie a knot after every straw. Join the ends of the string by tying them together. There, your toddler just made a beautiful straw necklace.

Squirt gun painting

For this activity, hang a canvas on a board or use a sketching pad. Fill a squirt gun with watercolor and let your kid spray the canvas randomly. You should consider mixing the colors to give the paint an appealingly unique look.

Palm painting

Have your toddler dip the palm of their hands in paint and put a print on a piece of canvas. You can have a whole pad full of your toddler's prints with a different color on each page. Apart from enhancing artistic skills, the activity provides a good source of toddlerhood memory. This method can also be used to make fingerprint flowers.

Making paper rainbow

What is more beautiful than using craft to teach science? Here is how. Give your kid a card with the rainbow image as control. Now give the toddler a set of colored paper strips. Let the toddler arrange the colors of the rainbow as observed on the control card. You can add more learning lessons like naming the colors in the correct order and gluing the strips on a placard and hanging them in your kid's room.

Spray paint craft

Avail a variety of spray paints. Write any word on a placard, cover the word with a tape such that the tape fits every letter, and can be read. Invite your toddler to spray paint the placard using different colors. Once done, remove the tapes to expose the word you had written.

Chapter 8: Movement the Montessori way

There is often a lot of emphasis placed on the idea that children should be moving frequently to help keep their weight to a healthy level. Although, it isn't just their body weight but also their brain development that should be considered when we encourage children to move more. In relation to the Montessori approach, the freedom to move around applies more to them having the opportunity to roam around their classroom and home, both inside and outside.

Free Movement and Sensory Exploration

For a Montessori child to be able to move around freely in their environment, careful consideration must be applied so that there is some space—even if your home space is confined—and it is safe.

Earlier in this guide, we mentioned the importance of keeping a clean and simple environment. One main reason for this is so the child can move and explore freely. Everything that exists within the environment ought to be there for a reason and not just for its own sake. To help your child to move around freely and to foster sensory exploration, please consider the following:

The environment is suitable for the child's height and size.

Things are reachable for the child. For instance, the shelves are low enough for them to take things off and put them back neatly without any strain.

Ideally, you want to create an environment that allows the development of the five senses (touch, smell, taste, sound and sight).

Please remember that while children are given the freedom to move around, they must also be able to abide by certain ground rules in order to develop a respect and appreciation for their environment.

Purposeful "Movement" Work

Even today, we still find educators who do not truly grasp the importance and connection between the intellectual mind and moving the physical body. What's profound about Montessori's findings is she discovered that it's **purposeful** movement (movement that's connected to what is being learned), which is the key. For instance, if you ask your child to go and collect ten twigs and bring them back to you, the child is learning to develop muscle memory through an intentional movement.

Integration of Montessori Materials

To encourage the child to be able to integrate Montessori Materials, you could consider sensorial materials three-part cards. They help a child become familiar with sensory materials and their names. For example, three-part cards contain a "control" card that is printed with a picture of a sensorial image on one side, and on the other side, it states the name of the image. This also has a positive impact on fine and gross motor skills as the child can carry out activities that involve "picture to object" or vice-versa. We will discuss this further shortly.

Benefits of fine and gross motor skills

It's essential to define the difference between fine and gross motor skills. Fine motor skills are what we make to move the small muscles, such as the hands and wrists. So as a parent, you would be looking at how your child holds a pencil, how they use their utensils while they are eating, etc. Gross motor skills are what we use to make movements with all our muscles, limbs, and joints in a coordinated way. So, when children walk, jump, climb, skip, etc. they are using gross motor skills. Most of the time, gross motor skills relate to their core strength. For example, can they sit up straight? Do they have good control and coordination to run?

Below are some more benefits that fine and gross motor skills can offer your child.

Benefits of fine motor skills

Children learn to use tools such as scissors, crayons, chalk, pencils, etc. Fine motor skills enable them to cut food, draw, paint, and write, to name a few.

Children can perform essential tasks with more precision, like moving objects, reaching out for things, and grasping. For example, they can zip or button up a coat, write their names or sign them, and turn the pages of their favorite books!

Hand-eye coordination improves along with fine motor skills. As adults, such coordination allows us to drive cars, wash our hair, **etc.**

Children learn to develop their handwriting and draw pictures.

Children build self-esteem and confidence because they are developing their independence.

Benefits of gross motor skills

Children are healthy because they can move their bodies through exercise.

Brain development increases.

Children release energy through movement.

A child's self-esteem and confidence increase.

Children develop the skill of assessing risks, which in turn helps with decision-making as they grow older.

Learning Through Play

Playing comes naturally for most children. Even adults want the opportunity to play because it's so fundamental to our nature. It involves **not** setting goals, make-believe, having fun, and enjoying the present moment and spontaneity. Some playful activities have more potential to bring out the best in a child. Here are some examples:

Playing in the sand. When a child engages in this activity, they are enhancing their scientific learning and physical development. They are scooping up the sand, digging, sifting, and pouring. Essentially, they are finding out more about how things work (sand) and building their muscles and coordination. If they are playing in the sand with other children, then they are also learning about teamwork, social interaction and the importance of sharing.

Water play. Much like sand play, children are learning about the elements and how they work. They get to learn this in a safe environment, and they also get to learn about cause and effect—how there are consequences to actions.

Roleplay with dressing up. It is fun for children to have the freedom to put on dress-up clothes and use props such as "pretend" cooking, doctors and nurses' kits, scientist or detective kits. This provides them the opportunity to be anything from a bus driver, singer, shop assistant, fashion designer, inventor, or astronaut. This activity allows the child to start to make sense of the adult world, the roles played out in society, and they start to gain insight into what interests them. Also, when children dress up, it helps to remind them about self-care.

Playing with dolls or characters. This isn't just about girls playing with dolls. When children are encouraged to play with dolls or mini figures, such as lego, they are learning about social play, how to label feelings, expression, and of course, imagination.

Imaginative play helps a child to develop their literacy skills, intellectual reasoning, self-esteem and self-confidence. You only need to leave a child with a few random objects, and they will let their imagination do the rest. This should be encouraged for as long as possible during their childhood years. This will enable them to think creatively throughout life and also enhance their problem-solving skills.

Nature play. This type of play is healthy, encourages the child to have respect for nature and the environment overall. They also get to learn about biology and their curiosity becomes stimulated. If you let a child out into the great outdoors, their potential to learn and develop will magnify.

Play is one of the best ways a child can learn. Not only does play assist with formal learning later in childhood, but it also encourages scientific thinking. For children who are experiencing early years, play **plays** (pun intended) a pivotal role in childhood development for language, creativity, emotional intelligence and intellectual reasoning.

Play helps a child develop their social, emotional, physical, and intellectual skills. Playtime for the child might involve banging toys around as they stamp their feet or having two toys play out a scenario that resembles real life. Children choose to play and doing so helps with developing their self-esteem because they start to realize what they can do. They can also develop life skills because often they will imitate the actions and behaviors of adults around them. They also develop their concentration skills due to having so much fun playing that they are completely immersed. If your child is playing with both adults and children, it will help them become socially confident as they grow older.

Here are some ways your child can develop motor skills through playing:

Physically playing by running, throwing, peddling, rolling around, and climbing. These activities will help with gross motor skills.

To encourage your child to grow their fine motor skills, why not let them button up their shirt or zip up their coat? Writing is excellent for encouraging children to put down their thoughts and feelings in the written word; it will do wonders for them. If they can write, perhaps they could start to write down things they are grateful for daily. This also encourages positivity and happiness.

For the Newborn

Give your newborn containers to play with

Play peek-a-boo with your baby

Hide and seek

Play music and clap

Read books

Let them see themselves in the mirror

For the Infant:

Three-colored spheres (previously discussed)

Dancing and singing

Object performance using sensorial materials such as three-part cards

Interlocking rings—This involves three or four rings that are interlocked. This is an excellent holding toy.

They could stick and separate hair rollers

Play with stickers and felt

Stack toy utensils: stack and knock over (empty) cups

DIY finger paints

Play with giant felt pieces

Pincer grip: pull fabric pieces from a tissue box

For the Toddler

Helping when you're washing up—If you make this fun, they'll get into the habit of doing this even when they grow older.

Singing and playing musical instruments

Playing ball games

Weaving and sewing

Walking heel to toe on a line—an excellent way to enhance motor skills and focus

Playing with dough, painting pictures and drawing—These activities are still fun even for adults!

Playing make-believe or "let's pretend"

Building blocks—especially Lego!

Playing with sand and water—This activity will allow the child to understand that water isn't solid.

Chapter 9: How to Create a Montessori Environment at Home

Montessori education does not have to be limited to classrooms. In fact, proponents of this method advise parents to continue it at home. This includes making small changes both to the physical home environment and the thinking of the parents.

Creating a Montessori environment at home does not require a dramatic change in home life and structure. It is simple but makes profound effects on the child's development.

Simplify the environment

Spaces for children are often bright and filled with various knick-knacks, thinking that the more toys available for children, the smarter they become. That's not always true. Too much stimulation can be bad for children.

Montessori spaces can be viewed as minimalist. The colors are neutral in order to create a soothing environment. It is not too busy with large prints and very bright colors. The soothing environment promotes concentration.

Materials are much less compared to non-Montessori spaces. There are fewer toys and décor on the walls. A small shelving unit is present. There are 2-3 shelves with a few items on each self. There are plenty of spaces in between the toys.

If the child already has many toys, put some in storage for later use. Choose the ones that are most suited to the child's age and current interests to put on the shelves.

By keeping the number of choices small, it will be easier to observe what the child is really interested in. Observe. If the child has not touched a once-favorite toy for an entire week, that toy may have been outgrown or no longer suited to the child's needs. Put it in storage.

Change the toys regularly. This can help keep the child interested without having to buy new toys every time.

Everything has its own place

Again, this is at the core of Montessori. Have a place for every item so that the child knows where to get it and where to put it back. This caters to the child's natural inclination for order and repetition. It also gives them a sense of security when they know they can expect something to be in the same place every time they go to it. Predictability is also calming for the child.

Open spaces

Embrace open spaces. Parents don't have to fill every nook and cranny with educational toys and books. Montessori environments has open spaces where children can work. Open spaces allow for movements, something many young children enjoy doing.

Accessible

Keep things low enough for children to reach. Shelves holding toys and materials should be within the child's reach. The tables and chairs should be low enough so that small children can sit down and get up from on their own.

Incorporate nature

A large window that lets in natural light is a good thing. The child can observe the changing light or observe the rain through the window. The child may also be allowed to have access to the window (ensure safety with proper locks and barriers to avoid accidents) to observe the outside world.

Plants on the windowsill can add a touch of nature to the Montessori space. This can even be used to be part of the Montessori activities such as Practical Life.

Carefully choose the toys

Toys do not necessarily have to be all educational toys. Parents should consider what effect the toys can have on the child. It should depend on the age and the developmental level of the child. For example, babies should be given toys that promote development of gross motor skills. A few baby-friendly toys that help develop fine motor skills are also good.

Toys that stimulate open-ended play are also appropriate to provide for the child.

Cozy

One of the most basic aspects to consider is comfort. The Montessori space can be everything but won't be effective if the child isn't comfortable being in it.

The Montessori space should be a place for the child to rest and relax while still developing skills and learning.

Chapter 10: Toddling

As your little human develops from being entirely dependent on you to becoming increasingly autonomous, more worries and decisions crop up. You want to protect your little child from all sadness and negativity, but it's also your job to prepare them for life, and, as we explored in the previous chapter, the two often don't go hand-in-hand.

Just as you were getting the hang of having a baby around, your baby up and grew. Now you have a child who is a newly minted walker and talker. They recall a whole slew of questions. Is it okay to tell little Norah no, or will it damage them self-esteem? Should you start letting them have a say in some of the family decisions? How soon should they potty train? Will they be psychologically damaged if you let them keep sucking them thumb? What should you do if they throw a tantrum in public? Should you always give them what they want whenever you can? What if they hate you?

A modern wave of parenting fads would have you believe that you should treat children as equals, that their self-esteem is fragile, and shame on you if you don't show that you care about every thought and feeling that enters their minds and leaves their mouths. There is some validity to it but be wary when someone tells you that something seemingly small—like not giving your child a choice between peanut butter or ham for lunch—is going to screw them up.

While child abuse and neglect have been found to ruin a child's self-esteem, no evidence supports the idea that you should let your kid walk all over you and be a demanding brat. In fact, a toddler **needs** boundaries and restrictions to feel secure, healthy, and happy.

The Brain Development of a Toddler

Between the first and second year, a toddler's brain increases the number of synapses, forming rapid connections and undergoing what's commonly referred to as a vocabulary explosion. As myelination (a process that allows nerve impulses to move more quickly) increases, the brain becomes capable of greater complexity. For example, a two-year-old will begin to form an understanding of their own self-awareness and begin to use personal pronouns.

By three years old, a child's brain will have twice as many synapses as an adult brain and show great plasticity. A three-year-old child will begin to understand more complex concepts like past and present and cause and effect.

Don't let a toddler's large number of synapses fool you, though. Toddlers' brains work in fundamentally different ways from adult humans, says Marguerite Lamb (SOURCE). For instance, when Norah wants a banana, but you don't have a banana to give her, she won't understand why she can't have a banana even when you explain the logical reasons why you can't give her one. The synapses in their frontal lobe haven't adequately developed at this point in their life for them to understand and accept such an abstract idea.

Toddlers, in their new sense of self-awareness, are self-centered and irrational. They can't help it; it's how their brains are wired thus far. They are not mini adults, and it's necessary that you understand that if you want to make it past the toddler stage without screwing them up.

Things That Will Screw Up a Toddler

There are several obvious things that will screw up your toddler. Leaving toxic chemicals within reach, for instance, can be detrimental. Neglect is another. Rather obviously, abuse is another one. Remember that book A Child Called It, by Dave Pelzer? For those of you who don't know, it's a memoir about the mind games an alcoholic mother plays with her youngest son, later nearly killing him.

The Mini-Adult Thinking

According to child psychologist Dr. Thomas Phelan, creator of the program 1-2-3 Magic, one of the more effective punishments for a toddler is to put them in time out. Remove them from the furniture, place them in a corner, on a chair, in their bedroom, or any predetermined spot, and tell them they have to sit there for three minutes—a minute for each year of their life. This is not when you talk to them about your reasons. They're too young to understand the talking, but they will learn to understand that the consequence of not obeying you is to have to sit on the boring chair in the corner. They will also learn something more valuable: when you say no, you mean it. When a toddler understands that your no is unchangeable, they will learn that throwing a tantrum isn't an effective tactic for getting what they want.

A common mistake that parents make when disciplining is that they don't control their own emotions. When you lose your temper at your child, you abdicate your emotional responsibility and give it to the youngest and least mature person in your household. Why would you do that? Well, you certainly don't mean to.

Overstimulation

There's been a craze among middle class American parents to expose their children to any number of things from pre-literacy Mandarin tutoring to yoga to media-based educational programming. But is there any benefit from it? Perhaps some, but many times this comes with a price—and we don't necessarily mean a money price. As babies grow into toddlers, they become better at blocking out certain stimuli and reacting to others, but when they get tired or bombarded with too many things at once, their skills are often not equal to the task of sorting everything out. They get overwhelmed.

Overstimulated toddlers might avoid eye contact to diminish the amount of stimulation they are receiving, crawl under the table, be disobedient, behave more irrationally than is normal for a toddler, cry, or even have a total meltdown. They react this way because they don't yet have the language to express the way they're feeling.

Toddlers need stimulation in order to learn and grow, but when they've had too much stimulation and can't take it anymore, it can lead to behavior problems that, when repeated over the course of months and years, can become habits that are difficult to get rid of. Behavior problems that result from constant over-stimulation can have long-term negative effects on your relationship with your child.

Keep screen time to a minimum with your toddler, as the stimulation of TV programming and games on the computer can also over-stimulate your child while also encouraging them to be a passive watcher rather than engaging their brain. Instead, make time to play with your toddler, as playing and talking with them is hugely pivotal to their healthy development.

Catherine Crawford, author of French twist observed in her own two children that when they paused their imaginary game to watch TV, they were more contentious with each other once they returned to their play. It was harder for them to get along, and it took a while for them to get the hang of playing together without fighting.

Things That Won't Screw Up a Toddler

The things that won't screw up your toddler are more numerous than you might imagine. We will explore below a few of the things parents fear might mess their kids up, but which are in fact good for them and are key to developing a healthy concept of self and the world around them.

Saying No

Telling your toddler, no won't ruin them. Often, children do things, say things, or ask for things they're not allowed to have in order to test the boundaries. Of course, little Max wants you to give in and buy him the giant Lego set, but he's not going to hate you if you don't. He might tell you that he hates you, but that is a completely different thing from actually hating you.

Consistency in your naysaying will save both you and your child time bargaining and cajoling and help them to move on to other subjects. When a child knows that no means no, it saves both of you time and hassle, and can lead to doing and saying things that can nurture a loving relationship.

Be careful of saying no too often and without reason. Some parents fall into the habit of saying no without any real reason. Davy, a father of six kids under the age of ten, admits that sometimes he says no simply because he's tired and left alone, even though he knows that he should say yes. "When the boys want to play touch football in the yard, I know I should play with them and be a good role model for them. Not every time, of course, but more often than I do."

If the kids want to go play in the street, street danger is a legitimate reason to tell them not to. If the kids want to play in the yard and ask you to come out with them and there isn't a reason that this will screw them up in any way, say yes.

There are absolutely times when you need to say yes. When Max wants to play trucks in the yard, and you can't think of a reason why you're telling him no other than that you're the parent and you said so, that might be an indication that you should be saying yes instead. After all, interactive playtime is significant to a toddler's development.

Discipline

A toddler is not too young to receive punishment for wrongdoing. In fact, the sooner you teach them that their actions have consequences, the less you will have to discipline them in the future.

One of the keys to effectively disciplining a toddler is to choose a punishment that fits the crime. Grounding a toddler doesn't make any sense. The point of discipline is to teach Norah that her actions have consequences, and what she does affects what happens to her. If she scribbles with markers all over her bedroom wall, hand her a scrub brush and help her clean the wall off. The most effective kinds of consequences are natural consequences. When she realizes that scrubbing the crayon off the wall is hard, she'll think twice before coloring it next time she takes her crayons out to make art.

Mona used grounding as her primary means of disciplining her three-year-old. She'd tell him to stop throwing his toys, and when he didn't listen to her, she'd tell him that he was not allowed to watch TV for a week. While this strategy might work on an older child, a toddler won't understand the correlation between throwing toys and no TV. When it comes to disciplining toddlers it's best to keep the punishment in line with the crime, as well as to dish it out immediately. Rather than grounding a child for throwing toys, try a time out or taking away the toys for a day.

Not giving a constant barrage of choices

A toddler doesn't have abstract reasoning skills. Particularly if you live in the upper middle-class suburbs, helicopter parents, who constantly hover over their kids protecting them from any negative emotions and offering them a giant spread of lunch meat from which to choose their lunch, are becoming strangely normal. These parents, out of fear of having their child experience hurt and disappointment, strive to give their children the best they can always. No sacrifice is too big. This sounds noble, but what they don't realize is that giving a child a constant barrage of choices, like more than one dinner option in case they don't like something, either runs the risk of over-stimulating them or it reinforces their already very selfish worldview.

A child whose parents cater to their every whim doesn't learn how to deal with their frustration and disappointment. Also, a child who is presented with a steady stream of choices runs of risk of becoming over-stimulated and having a meltdown.

The person who spread the myth that children have fragile self-esteem that needs to be protected at all costs has clearly never seen a toddler. A toddler is incredibly self-absorbed. When you give them a lot of choices, you're reinforcing their view of their-self as the center of the universe. Of course, there is nothing inherently wrong with giving a kid some choices. Good decision-making is obviously a skill that you want to teach him, but don't take it to ridiculous heights, or they will get overwhelmed and then start to assume that they are always entitled to having a choice in everything.

Delayed Gratification

Patience can be taught as early as infancy, but it's definitely not too late to learn as a toddler.

One way that you can teach your child to be patient is to let them pick out a treat when they go shopping with you, but don't let them eat it as soon as they get to the car. Instead, have them save it for their snack time later. A child who learns how to be patient early on in life will be a more patient adult. The problems that a lot of American children are having in school and at home stem from not being taught how to have patience.

Learning the art of delayed gratification can be one of the most useful, long-lasting lessons you can teach your child to keep from screwing them up.

Chapter 11: Common Parenting Mistakes when Training Toddlers

In this chapter, you will be introduced to some of the mistake's parents make when training their little children. If you find yourself susceptible to any of these mistakes, you should navigate around them with better strategies founded on an basic principle that will be shown in the latter part of this study guide.

Distorting the Routine

Toddlers work at their best capacities when the routine is predictable. Whether it is sleep, food or alertness, it is your duty to know the daily activities of your toddlers and to make them repetitive. Some parents don't know the circadian rhythm of their toddlers. This is the internal clock in the brain of a person. It measures the consistencies in the sleepiness and activeness of a person at regular intervals. As a parent, you should monitor the consistencies in the sleep- and wake-cycle of your toddler, as well as yours.

Using a Method of Coercion

One of the parental attitudes that experts sorely disapprove of is one in which the parent pressures or coerces toddlers into doing an action. It doesn't matter whether the action your toddler is coerced into doing is bad or not, pressuring your toddlers is a vice that has lifetime detriments on them. Coercion has terrible effects on your toddler's eating attitude.

Modest Method of Coercion

Bribery

Smart parents find a way around things. This is detrimental to the toddler's behavior. They often apply a modest method of coercion by promising the toddler a reward of a favorite food after eating a disliked food.
According to psychologist Dr. Leann Birch of the Pennsylvania State University, if the promised food is dessert, it makes the toddler value dessert more than more nutritious foods like vegetables and meats.

Serving Toddlers Big Food Items

According to the **American Dietetic Association** in Chicago, parents tend to serve children food items that are not compatible with their stomachs. When the food is relatively big to the child, they feel intimidated and frustrated to complete the seemingly heavy task of eating a huge meal.

Succumbing to Your Toddler's Denial of New Foods

This should not be mistaken for coercion. It simply means some parents make the mistake of not trying the law of consistency when introducing new foods to their toddlers.

As Dr. Birch notes, it may require between 10 to 15 times of presentation before a toddler can finally adopt a new food.

Dr. Jean Skinner, another reputable dietitian at the University of Tennessee, also posits that to fulfill the necessary criterion of your toddlers eating a variety of foods, there is a need for you to consistently offer a variety of foods.

According to Satter, a display of hysterical happiness when the toddler finally accepts to eat a new food may also make the child avoid the food eventually.

Intolerance to Messy Mealtimes

Excessiveness is when you expect a toddler to keep all the table manners you have acquired in the social world.

Many parents think taste is the only way food is enjoyed. While this is true for an adult, it isn't the case for a toddler. According to experts in Food and Nutrition Science, there are many sensory organs that children use to enjoy food. They tend to enjoy the food more when they play with it and get themselves all messy.

Many parents who express sore displeasure to these messy eating manners have the tendency to distort the enjoyment toddlers have when eating.

For children, forget about table manners and let them eat. The nutrition they consume takes more importance than whether they eat neatly or not.

Having seen some of the mistakes that parents make when training toddlers, it is beneficial to also see some general consequences of these mistakes.

Rigidly Rebuking Your Toddler's Mistakes

Correcting mistakes that are made is necessary, but when the scrutiny becomes intense, you may be digging a very deep pitfall for your toddlers in the future. Parents who take an extreme correctional approach to the mistakes of their children usually have the conception that this will make them better and perfect. When the child eventually grows into an adult and makes mistakes, their sense of personal worth takes a dent. they punish their-self by subjecting their-self to self-flagellating thoughts, which is a gateway to depression. they take a rigid approach to correcting themselves. In extreme cases, they may resort to self-harm. Other significant areas where parents often make mistakes are eating habits and toilet manners.

CONCLUSION

I hope you find this book a helpful resource to guide you in teaching self-care to your young child. There's little in life that is more satisfying than observing the feeling of content on a child's face when mastering a new skill.

One of the greatest impacts of the Montessori Teaching Method, chiefly during the early learning experience, is the concentration on hands-on learning. The stresses are on actual rather than intangible learning, as students make efforts on activities that instruct language, math, culture, and practical life lessons. Teachers motivate students to focus on errands, and they deject students from disturbing one another, permitting children to concentrate on activities until they are appropriately mastered.

The next step is to map out your action plan to follow these suggested tips and carry out the informative guidelines to set up a Montessori-inspired setting. As this can be done in the comfort of your home, it will help you raise your toddler efficiently on your own. Most parents think that homeschooling is an impossible concept in today's world where even for preschool readiness, they have opened pre-preschools! Though you must be thinking otherwise after reading this guidebook.

A properly implemented Montessori curriculum and scientific approach can be highly effective in producing men capable of reasoning and problem solving but independently efficient in their work and deriving pleasure from it. After being raised as a Montessori toddler, this sort of mindset shows that education is not just for task completion, but it is for life and is life itself. The Montessori toddlers are socially confident, emotionally stable human beings with spiritual love and a sense of responsibility present at their very core.

Ultimately, if you want to take things further, you can consider the minimalist lifestyle. You do not have to jump into it with both feet. We have provided proven methods and examples in this manual to help you decide if the minimalist lifestyle works for you.

And finally, if you still are worried about what you should do and what you shouldn't, how to identify any delays, and what to expect in terms of their developmental milestones, use this detailed guide to help you. This has all the information you will possibly need to track their physical, speech, cognitive, and sensory development. So, use it wisely and act like a responsible and good parent.

Enjoy the journey!

DO YOU WANT MORE?

SCAN ME

CPSIA information can be obtained
at www.ICGtesting.com
Printed in the USA
LVHW081812010621
689062LV00015B/1704

9 781802 936797